CUM AS YOU ARE

while transforming your sex life

Rita J. Alexander

CONTENTS

INTRODUCTION

Regardless of how fulfilling things are in the room, we, as a whole, prefer to flavor things up from time to time. Yet, imagine a scenario where you could change your sexual coexistence with only a couple of basic changes.

We should envision briefly that a genie seems to make you an arrangement. On one condition, you can have all the cash you need: from the second you acknowledge his proposition, your sexual coexistence won't ever beat it as of now. Could you be all right with that? Or, on the other hand, could you need to hold out with the expectation that your sexual coexistence could one day move along? Many of us would need to pick the last option, which is OK; it simply implies you could profit from learning more about your sexuality. Luckily, that is where this synopsis comes in! Through these parts, we'll investigate some logical exploration that makes sense of how a setting can upgrade or hinder your sexual experience and why individuals are so unique regarding their degrees of want. You'll likewise learn:

Why male and female genitalia aren't generally so unique as you would suspect

How seeing a lion can demolish your sexual experience (yet not for the reasons you could think) and

Why disposing of your ladies' magazines will support your sex life.

"Well. The disappointing truth is we've been deceived — not purposely, it's nobody's shortcoming, yet. We recounted some unacceptable stories. For quite a long time in Western science and medication, ladies' sexuality was seen as Men's Sexuality Light —

fundamentally the equivalent yet not exactly as great."

"Be that as it may, to comprehend human sexuality, conduct alone will not get you there. Attempting to comprehend sex by seeing the way of behaving is like attempting to figure out adoration by taking a gander at a couple's wedding picture . . . what's more, their legal documents."

Per their "double control model," the sexual reaction system in our minds comprises a couple of available parts — a sexual gas pedal and sexual brakes — and those parts answer general classes of sexual feelings, including genital sensations, visual sensations, excitement, and close to the home setting. Also, the awareness of every part shifts from one individual to another."

"We as a whole are made of similar parts, however in every one of us, those parts are coordinated in a special way that changes over our life expectancy."

"It turns out what makes the biggest difference isn't the parts you are made of or how they are coordinated, yet how you feel about those parts."

CHAPTER 1: OUR BODIES ARE QUITE SO UNIQUE AS YOU WOULD NATURALLY SUSPECT...

Assuming you analyze the male and female life systems, our disparities could appear as though we're principally described. Furthermore, where we, in all actuality, do have shared characteristics, sometimes it simply appears bizarre because men have areolas. All things considered, for what reason do they require them? On a female body, we can figure out their motivation; female areolas assist moms with supporting their infants. In any case, how are men expected to manage them? Indeed, the response isn't very odd as you would suspect! That is because each individual is shaped with a similar fundamental body part; those parts simply revamp themselves from one individual to another through an interaction known as homology. This is the carefully guarded secret: for the initial six weeks of pregnancy, all babies have indistinguishable tissue. Whether or not that baby will grow up to have male, female, or intersex genitalia, everybody begins with a similar genital tissue.

Furthermore, regardless of how that embryo later creates, that tissue is additionally unquestionably delicate to excitement. That is additionally why male bodies have areolas: since everybody begins with a similar essential arrangement of parts, all hatchlings structure areolas. A lot later, their genitalia is created in the belly and assigned to them as male. In any case, the distinctions aren't simply tracked down in male and female privates. Truth be told, each lady's vagina is extraordinary, and no two are framed the very same way.

Sadly, be that as it may, vaginas are carefully restored for sexual entertainment to make the labia (or lips) less noticeable. This frequently gives individuals a ridiculous picture of what a vagina should resemble. Yet, whether you're male or female, you ought to recall that all sizes and shades of the vagina are typical (the same length as these elements aren't impacted by a disease that causes you torment). Furthermore, the equivalent is valid for the clitoris! This piece of the female life system can change from the size of a pea to that of a smaller than usual pickle.

"The thinking went this way: Ladies' private parts are concealed between their legs, as though they needed to be covered up, while male private parts look ahead, so anyone might be able to see. Also, how could people's privates be different along these lines? On the off chance that you're a middle age anatomist, saturated with a sexual ethic of immaculateness, this is because of disgrace."

"Homology is additionally why both siblings will have areolas. Areolas on females are imperative to the endurance of practically all vertebrate species, including people (however a modest bunch of old well evolved creatures, like the platypus, don't have areolas, and on second thought simply spill milk from their midsections), so development constructed areolas in right at the earliest reference point of our fetal turn of events. It takes less energy to simply leave them there than to effectively smother them — and development is as languid as it can pull off — so the two guys and females have areolas. Same organic starting points — various capabilities."

"Not at all like the penis, the clitoris' one responsibility is sensation. The penis has four positions: sensation, infiltration, discharge, and pee."

"In any case, the hymen doesn't break and always stays broken, similar to some newness seal. On the off chance that a hymen tears or injuries, it recuperates. What's more, the size of a hymen doesn't differ relying upon whether the vagina has been infiltrated. Likewise, it for the most part doesn't drain. Any blood with the first entrance is more probable because of general vaginal tearing from the absence of grease than to harm to the hymen."

CHAPTER 2: GET TO KNOW YOUR SEXUAL PERSONALITY...

"Your focal sensory system (your mind and spinal line) is comprised of a progression of organizations of gas pedal and brakes — like the matching of your thoughtful sensory system ("gas pedal") and your parasympathetic sensory system ("brake"). The central understanding of the double control model that's valid for different parts of the sensory system should likewise be valid for the mind framework that directs sex: a sexual gas pedal and sexual brake. (Daniel Kahneman composed his own Nobel Prize-winning exploration of financial matters, "You realize you have created a hypothetical development when you can never again remake why you fizzled for such a long time to see the self-evident." So it was with Kahneman's possibility hypothesis, thus it is with the double control model. I stand prepared to send Erick and John huge natural product containers on the day the Nobel board of trustees starts thinking responsibly and perceives the significance of their knowledge.) So the double control model of sexual reaction, as the name suggests, comprises two sections:"

"Sexual Excitation Framework (SEF)."

"Sexual Hindrance Framework (SHF)."

"The short response is: Decrease your pressure, be friendly toward your body, and let go of the bogus thoughts regarding how sex is "assumed" to work, to make space in your life for how sex functions."

Not long after conceiving an offspring, one of my patients, Claudie, communicated that she genuinely wanted to have intercourse with her significant other. In any case, she delighted in pleasuring herself with a wand or vibrator, and she before long came to feel that something wasn't quite right about her absence of want to have penetrative sex. Was there? In no way, shape, or form! Here's why: you can consider the human mind to have a sexual gas pedal and a sexual break. Your cerebrum is incited to siphon those breaks any time it identifies a danger, genuine or envisioned. That implies that any upgrades — from an idea to a smell to your accomplice's clothing — can set off your mind to accept that sex is not an extraordinary thought right now, and you then bang on the breaks.

All in all, how does that work? Indeed, when in doubt, a sensory system that effectively sets off breaks is the most widely recognized justification for sexual hang-ups. For instance, a 2008 investigation of 226 ladies found that respondents who battled to become excited or just experienced excitement under excellent conditions experienced critical sexual nervousness that hindered their experience. Yet, these battles ought not to be a reason to worry; everybody's sexual breaks and gas pedals have various degrees of responsiveness, which is completely ordinary. These distinctions structure every individual's novel sexual character. For instance, one more of my patients, Natasha, griped that she had an exceptionally low sex drive. She additionally encountered no sensations of excitement while seeing her accomplice or considering them in dreams. Be that as it may, for her situation, it wasn't because she was restless about sex or skeptical of her accomplice. All things being equal, the issue was essential that Natasha has a soft sexual gas pedal, and it's not as a very special issue as you would naturally suspect. It implies that she doesn't answer as quickly to sexual excitement as others would, and consequently, she needs some additional chance to get ready.

Good and contemporary ways to deal with the appraisal of female sexuality are talked about. General methodologies, appraisal techniques, and models of female sexuality are coordinated inside the reasonable spaces of sexual ways of behaving, sexual reactions (want, energy, climax, and goal), and individual contrasts, including general and sex-explicit character models.

Sexual way of behaving

Research in female sexuality is fractionated. Huge commitments in specific regions, like an appraisal, treatment, or understanding of sexual peculiarities, have not prompted branch-off commitments in related regions. Reflecting on the field of human sexuality, the investigation of ladies' sexuality has missed the mark on an all-encompassing reasonable premise with which to look at, assess, and guide progressing research; subsequently, to essentially progress sexual science, it has been recommended that we should foster exhaustive speculations and develops that depict, make sense of, and anticipate sexual peculiarities. The current commitment talks about issues in evaluating female sexuality from the authoritative structure of ideas as opposed to measures. Here, I will give data on works of art and contemporary methodologies. The conversation is outlined inside the applied areas of sexual ways of behaving, sexual reactions (i.e., the sexual reaction cycle), and individual contrasts.

Albeit a sexual reaction cycle conceptualization, explicitly want fervor, climax, and goal as a significant second part in a functioning model of female sexuality. Even though there are huge and significant interrelationships among the stages, there is adequate information to recommend that each has one-of-a-kind viewpoints. The different elaboration of the stages may likewise explain the female sexual dysfunctions, as most Analytic and Factual Manual of Mental Issues analyze are presently conceptualized by phasic disturbance. As we consider the evaluation of each stage, we think about four "channels" for appraisal: physiological, mental, full of feeling, and conduct.

The resurgence in character research in the previous ten years and my line of mental examination urges us to analyze the job of individual contrasts in ladies' sexuality, the contemporary association of character structure, and the Large Five model, as well as physically relevant character factors, like sexual self-blueprint.

Sexual Reaction Cycle

As stated by Rosen and Beck, "a basic presumption hidden most conceptualizations of sexual reaction [and that is that] sexual excitement processes are probably going to follow an anticipated succession of occasions, and that a repeating example of physiological answering might be recognized". In any case, there has been conflict about the number and significance of each stage. Although advocated by Bosses and Johnson, the idea of phases of sexual commitment has early beginnings. As summed up, the number of stages has gone from two to four. The periods of want, level, and goal are conflictingly addressed. At the same time, a two-layered model of excitement energy process and a climax or quick post orgasm stage has been reliable. By and large, specialists have zeroed in on grasping fervor (or sexual excitement). Yet, more as of late, there have been comparable accentuations on characterizing the mental and conduct limits of sexual longing. A useful examination of the predecessors, issues, ways of behaving, and outcomes of the specific sexual trouble is generally normal. Although the last option is extremely helpful, one may not be guaranteed to acquire data from pretty much all the sexual reaction cycle periods.

CHAPTER 3: YOUR SEXUAL EXPERIENCE RELIES UPON THE SPECIFIC CIRCUMSTANCE

Does this story sound natural? Two individuals meet, have a ridiculously energized outlook on one another, and jump into an enthusiastic sentiment supercharged with sex. Yet, it's not well before the energy begins to wear off, and before their second over a year together, the blazes have subsided to a simple glint. Since this occurs so regularly, many individuals get the possibility that it's typical for their sexual experiences to burn out or for accomplices to lose interest in each other. In any case, that is not guaranteed to be valid. Truth be told, whether a sensation feels energizing or outright irritating is completely subject to the setting of your sexual experience. Furthermore, in the story depicted over, that setting is the straightforward entry of time. In any case, fortunately, the setting is abstract and tends to be controlled.

For instance, suppose you're feeling attractive, and your accomplice stimulates you. In that state of mind, this sensation presumably feels shivery and energizing. Be that as it may, on the off chance that you were focusing on something significant, you may be irritated or even irate. This simply demonstrates that the setting directs whether a specific sensation is pleasurable or disturbing and decides if you and your accomplice engage in sexual relations or not. Concentrates on a show that assumes that the state of mind is correct; nearly anything can feel suggestive. For instance, one review on guinea pigs explored different avenues regarding a little test embedded into the rodent's core accumbens, which is found profound inside the cerebrum. In an unbiased climate, the researcher had a go at animating the higher piece of the core, and the rodent answered with indications of uplifted interest. When the researcher animated the core's lower area, the rodent answered with evasion.

In any case, when the rodent was out of that unbiased climate and in one it saw as remarkably certain — a setting with various charming scents and no light — it as of now not made a difference what part of the core the researcher tried. However long it was in that pleasant climate, the rodent stayed blissful and locked in. Also, the equivalent is valid for people! Regardless of whether you appreciate tickling or agony in your stable climate, under the right conditions (like a climate that feels both protected and provocative), being whipped or tied up can feel sensual in any event.

"It's actually in the entirety of your different faculties, in addition to the fundamental five you learned in grade school. We've all accomplished it with chemoreception: Envision your vehicle has run out of fuel one mile from the service station, on a singing hot, sauna-damp day. You walk the mile through the sludgy air. You get to the cooling service station, chilled to 72 degrees, and it seems like a cold impact, a strong help from the intensity. Presently envision your vehicle running dry in a similar spot a half year after the fact, and it's a sharply cool, bitingly breezy day, and you walk a similar mile to the service station. That equivalent 72 degrees presently feels like a warmed broiler, a strong help from the difficult virus. Setting."

"Going against the norm. In an investigation of cocaine fiends, research members' mesolimbic frameworks answered pictures connected with cocaine that glimmered on a screen for 33 milliseconds. Assuming you asked them what they saw, they wouldn't have the option to tell you, because the pictures streaked too quickly to even consider being "seen" intentionally, yet illuminating the fiends' energy systems was sufficiently long. The examination subjects didn't know about having seen the pictures, yet their profound cerebrums answered."

Sexual Craving
10 years after Experts and Johnson's detailing proposing sexual fervor as the main period of the reaction cycle, Kaplan and Lief affirmed an extended model that started with sexual craving, and the term repressed sexual longing was authored for people who persistently neglected to start or answer sexual signs.

Problems of Sexual Craving repeated the psychoanalytic place of the drive as a profound natural power that would be communicated in either sexual or nonsexual outlets. It would then follow that any hindrance of want would be because of the oblivious constraint or cognizant concealment of inclinations for sexual contact. Regardless, such safeguards would emerge from intrapsychic clashes encompassing sexuality.

There are interactional models of want and ones that underline other, nondynamic mental cycles, for instance, features the job of sexual drive, seen as a naturally based source, and the person's social and mental endeavors to look for sexual excitement. Conversely, sexual inspiration, similar to craving or thirst, rises out of the cooperation of outer motivating forces (i.e., a sexual upgrade) and interior states (e.g., sexual hardship). Want is both a setting occasion and a result of sexual activity. At last, is a mental yearning for a sexual association attached to sexual fulfillment and relational relationship fulfillment (i.e., love) for the accomplice.

Biologic models of sexual craving are disputable and, as of now, underscore hormonal instruments. Information is generally steady for the vital (yet not adequate) job of androgens, most likely testosterone. For this model, most of the supporting information comes from men; Bancroft recommends that the event of unconstrained erections during rest are the social appearances of the androgen-based neurophysiological substrate of sexual longing; interestingly, erections with a dream or suggestive viewable signals are viewed as proof for androgen-free reactions.

Chemical sexual conduct connections for ladies are less clear, even though estrogen, progesterone, and androgen (testosterone) have been contemplated. Concerning impacts, some measure of estrogen is vital for typical vaginal oil, and receipt of estrogen substitution treatment after menopause might diminish the dangerous side effects (e.g., absence of oil, atrophic vaginitis) and permit sexual action or working to continue healthy. Interestingly, progesterone may make an inhibitory difference. At last, testosterone might straightforwardly affect sexual working; both Bancroft and Wu and Schreiner-Engel, Schiavi, Smith, and White have found positive connections between testosterone levels and recurrence of masturbation and vaginal reactions to sensual improvements. In investigations of people for whom estrogen treatment was not viable for postmenopausal side effects, testosterone organization worked on sexual craving and related results. In concentrating on 19 oral preventative clients, plasma levels of free testosterone were related to self-report proportions of sexual longing, sexual considerations, and expectation of sexual activity.

Nonetheless, a fascinating and more straightforward trial of the speculation that testosterone is connected with sexual perceptions was disconfirmed; utilizing a particular consideration (dichotic tuning in) task, At long last, looking at 17 ladies who met Symptomatic and Factual Manual of

Mental Problems models for loss of want with 13 solid, physically dynamic ladies. Blood tests were drawn each 3-4 days for one monthly cycle and were dissected for testosterone, estradiol, progesterone, prolactin, and luteinizing chemicals. No distinctions between the gatherings were found, and subgroup investigations (e.g., examination of ladies with a deep-rooted shortfall of want versus those with procured loss of want) were likewise disconfirming. As of now, it is hazy whether physiologic measures and hormonal examinations, specifically, are helpful physiologic signs of sexual craving.

Sexual Energy
Either physical or psychological sexual feelings can start sexual energy. The real changes with sexual energy are significant. The overall physiologic reactions are far-reaching vasocongestion, shallow or profound, and myotonia, with one or the other intentional or compulsory muscle compressions. Different changes remember increments for a pulse and circulatory strain and more profound, faster breath. For ladies, sexual energy is additionally described by the presence of vaginal oil, created by vasocongestion in the vaginal walls, prompting liquid seepage. Different changes incorporate a slight growth of the clitoris and uterus with engorgement. The uterus likewise ascends ready, with the vagina extending and swelling out. Maximal vasocongestion of the vagina delivers a clogged orgasmic stage in the lower 33% of the vaginal barrel. As examined later, people may not know about the physiologic impressions of excitement; regardless of whether they are, their influences might be concurrent. In this manner, in the accompanying conversation, we think about both positive effects, like excitement, and negative effects, for example, uneasiness, which might connect with sexual fervor. Thought of negative influences is pertinent as some (e.g., tension) are key in hypothetical models of sexual fervor challenges or dysfunctions.

Excitement and other positive feelings Studies have tended to the physiological and emotional parts of excitement. Albeit the previously mentioned depiction notes vasocongestion and oil as the substantial overwhelming reactions, psychophysiological research has generally comprised of proportions of vaginal vasocongestion (i.e., vaginal pulse amplitude [VPA], vaginal blood volume [VBV]) utilizing the vaginal plethysmograph. Other genital estimations (like those for grease) have not arisen, are temperamental, or are not delicate to changes in excitement. As a physiological mark of sexual excitement, it is as yet muddled what these vaginal signs address and whether they are analogs of particular vascular cycles. In any case, there is proof of their focalized legitimacy. For instance, VPA and VBV are fit for distinguishing bunch contrasts (e.g., contrasts in as outright degrees of excitement between ladies with and those without sexual dysfunctions) and responsiveness to exploratory circumstances (e.g., novel openness and adjustment to sensual improvements, contrasts between suggestive versus nonerotic upgrades). Of the two measures, different information propose that VPA is the more delicate and solid genital measure, especially given its lack of care toward nervousness summoning boosts.

The development of arousability is vital to grasp the mental and emotional parts of sexual fervor in ladies. Bancroft indicates that arousability is a mental aversion to outside sexual prompts. He proposes that high arousability suggests upgraded insight, mindfulness, handling of sexual signals, and the substantial reactions of sexual fervor. This model tries to interface mental full of feeling reactions with control of genital and fringe signs of sexual energy through a neurophysiological substrate for sexual excitement. Luckily, one of the psychometrically most grounded self-report measures for female sexuality is one that additionally taps sexual arousability, the Sexual Arousability Record (SAI) by Hoon). On this 28-thing measure, ladies rate their sexual excitement for various sensual and unequivocal sexual ways of behaving. Both the clinical handiness and the force of the instrument are probable because of the significant advances that were taken in the scale development and approval process, including choosing things that proved focalized legitimacy with standard factors like ladies' attention to physiological changes during sexual excitement (e.g., vaginal oil, areola erection, sex flush, bosom enlarging, solid strain), evaluations of fulfillment with responsiveness, and sexual conduct measures. The action tests a scope of individual and joined forces sensual and sexual ways of behaving; our psychometric examinations show that the SAI tests the accompanying spaces: excitement related to erotica (e.g., writing or photography) and masturbation, tempting exercises (e.g., passionate kissing, being stripped down), body touching by a male accomplice, oral-genital and genital feeling, and intercourse.

CHAPTER 4: STRESS IS A SEX-EXECUTIONER

Our feeling of excusing society is awkward with Feels. Our way of life says that on the off chance that the stressor isn't directly before us, then, at that point, we have no obvious explanation to feel worried thus, we ought to simply remove it. Subsequently, many people's concept of "stress the executives" is either to kill all stressors or to simply unwind, as though stress can be switched off like a light switch. Our way of life is so awkward with Feels that we might try and steady individuals who've recently been in a fender bender, keeping their bodies from traveling through this regular cycle; this benevolent clinical mediation has the undesirable outcome of catching overcomers of horrible injury in the freeze, which is the way PTSD gets traction in a survivor's cerebrum.

However, can we just be real? We, as a whole, knew that generally, correct? What's more, assuming you want any additional assistance in envisioning it, we should simply envision that your accomplices jumped into your work for a quick in and out. You two are mishandling your direction down the lobby, searching for the most readily accessible secret spot, when you run into your boss out of nowhere and catch a hard, censuring gaze. The sort of gaze says she understands what you're doing and is cautioning you not to attempt it. Also, from that point forward, it would be really difficult to attempt to recover the mindset.

That is because pressure makes sex seem the ugliest thing on the planet. Sadly, you can't place your body's pressure reaction on hold or rush through the method involved with de-pressurizing. We even see this reaction in the animals of the world collectively because, for example, assuming a gazelle is being pursued by a lion, they have three choices: run, battle, or pretend to be dead. Also, regardless of their choice and whether it assists them with making due, their difficulties aren't finished. They'll keep encountering indications of stress like full-body quakes or fits long after the lion is no more.

These are good side effects of pressure leaving the body, known as de-pressurizing or finishing the pressure reaction cycle. Also, the equivalent is valid for you. So, even if you're not being pursued by a lion, the pressure of your work, family, or connections can, in any case, chase you down and leave you shaking. Furthermore, attempting to engage in sexual relations while going through the pressure interaction is a horrendous thought since you will not have the option to appreciate it until the cycle is finished. All in all, what is it that you do if you have any desire to rush through the cycle and begin having a good time once more? Indeed, you can't rush the cycle, yet you can attempt a few trustworthy sources for communicating your pressure that might be useful to it sooner. For instance, you can deliver strain through workout, rest, loosening up in the manner which causes you to feel generally great, or in any event, crying or shouting.

While these outlets work for many people, the cycle might be somewhat more convoluted for those who have experienced a sexual injury. Numerous survivors keep on feeling worried in any physically charged circumstance long after the risk is finished. Thus, assuming you've had to deal with a horrible encounter and your sense in any sexual circumstance is to essentially put on an act of being dead, that is typical. However, sadly, that can likewise drag out your recuperation pattern, which implies that it will take more time for you to track down a conclusion. Also, until you do, all things considered, you'll see practically any sexual circumstance as undermining. Notwithstanding, it is feasible to quiet down and achieve a feeling of harmony while attempting to engage in sexual relations, and rehearsing care can assist with that.

Enthusiastic love, characterized as a deep yearning for association with another, comprises three parts: mental (e.g., meddlesome reasoning or distraction with the accomplice), profound (fascination, and particularly physical allure, for the accomplice), and conduct viewpoints (e.g., endeavors to keep up with actual closeness to the accomplice, endeavors to help the accomplice). The action is corresponded, however, not covering important proportions of sexual longing and energy (e.g., interest in participating in sex with the accomplice, sensations of sexual fervor, appraisals of sexual fulfillment). Besides, ladies who have a positive perspective on themselves as sexual people and their capacity to turn out to be physically excited likewise report more significant levels of enthusiastic love and more heartfelt contributions.

Negative influences might disable energy; by and large, nervousness has been the estimated component in numerous hypotheses of excitement shortages. Psychodynamic theories accentuate fears of phallic-forceful motivations, mutilation, contention, or depraved object decisions. More vital to contemporary perspectives, Wolpe was quick to underline nervousness-based disability of physiologic reactions. In his view, the thoughtful movement normal for nervousness represses the nearby (i.e., genital) parasympathetic action liable for the underlying periods of sexual energy (i.e., erection for men and, probably, lubrication and vasocongestion for ladies). At first, proposed to make sense of male excitement shortages, the model has been applied less agreeably to ladies. There is minimal trial support for the dispute that the beginning stages of sexual excitement in ladies are principally parasympathetic or that tension will hinder the physiologic reactions of sexual excitement (even though uneasiness preexposure will impact verbal reports of emotional excitement.

Useless attentional cycles and negative influences have been the center of mental hypotheses of energy deficiencies. Experts and Johnson proposed two parts: "spectatoring" (i.e., attentional interruption as the person "watches" for their sexual answering) and pessimistic assumptions that the substantial reaction (e.g., erection) will be insufficient. Tension about execution disappointment (i.e., the shortfall of the physiologic reactions of fervor) then, at that point, happens. Once more, male sexual answering is typically the model for this model.

A covering, albeit more point-by-point, model is Barlow's. At the point when a positive, useful sexual reaction (e.g., an erection) would be normal, men with sexual troubles prove physiologic, mental, and profound qualities that lead to erectile disappointment. For instance, the information demonstrates that men with erection hardships underreport their degrees of sexual excitement (comparative with the extent of genuine erectile reaction) whenever questioned, concentrate on nonerotic instead of suggestive signals, and report pessimistic (discouraged) sentiments and an absence of command over their sexual reactions. This useless cycle is repeated and "gotten to the next level" (i.e., the broken individual turns out to be significantly more capable of zeroing in on some unacceptable parts of the sexual setting — the results of not playing out, the continuation of erectile deficiency). Subsequently, the singular comes to stay away from sexual settings later on.

Most of Barlow's tension and mental interruption model information comes from male members. At the point when the model has been analyzed, ladies (normally female students or, maybe, ladies enlisted from the local area) addressing "utilitarian" and "useless" bunches are tried in psychophysiology research centers. Ladies are given upgrades, generally, tapes, addressing tension-inciting, nonpartisan, or sexual arrangements. Vaginal measures, as well as self-reports of general or genital excitement, are recorded. In the trial of the physiologic impacts of tension, the information has, by and large, shown that genital excitement isn't hindered by uneasiness. Utilizing individualized, tension-inciting audiotaped situations, for instance, tracked down that genital excitement (VBV) expanded during the nervousness-inciting condition, albeit the levels were not generally so high as those accomplished during a sensual verbal boost. Gorzalka found that preexposure with a tension-inciting tape (e.g., a compromised removal), as opposed to an unbiased tape, worked with VBV reactions during the resulting review of suggestive scenes for the two ladies with and without sexual dysfunctions. This impact, preexposure to a tension inciting improvement expanding the ensuing VBV during erotica, has also been recreated. Different information disconfirming both the Bosses and Johnson and the Barlow conceptualizations is that by Laan, Everard, van Arnhold, and Agitator. They observed that VPA was higher (as opposed to lower) under trial "request" conditions (i.e., "Attempt to become as physically excited as conceivable inside 2 min and attempt to keep up with it however long you can. Your degree of sexual excitement will be recorded") interestingly, no interest conditions. Taken together, this information proposes that these past conceptualizations might be less significant (if applicable by any means) for ladies, as they validate neither the excitement processes (they might be predominately thoughtful instead of parasympathetic) nor speculated systems (e.g., execution interest).

Consequently, we consider tension and a wide band of influences that might be pertinent to segregating energy processes for evaluation. By the way, we note that the DSM-IV gives no hints regarding the heading of appraisal and generally excludes emotional models for excitement jumble in ladies. Interruption of a dominating physiologic reaction (lubrication and enlarging of the private parts) until the "culmination of sexual activity" is viewed as pathognomic, and this aggravation needs to result in all things considered "checked trouble" or "relational trouble."

Sexual uneasiness, or related terms, has been utilized to name scales that extensively contrast satisfaction and expectation. We likewise note that, instead of purpose recently distributed measures, numerous specialists usually foster their sexual uneasiness scales by adding a rating scale (e.g., a scale going from 0 [no nervousness at all] to 6 [extremely restless, apprehensive, or tense]) to a progressive conduct system, for example, the Bentler posting. A system much like the last option was E. Hoon's change of the SAI to the SAI — extended adaptation (SAI-E). She characterized uneasiness as a pessimistic sensation of pressure or apprehension. She utilized the SAI things yet changed the anchors for the rating scale (7-point Likert scale going from — 1 [relaxing] to 5 [extremely nervousness provoking]). Amazingly, in a legitimacy study, the SAI and the uneasiness evaluations on the SAI-E were uncorrelated. Yet, the tension evaluations were conversely connected with reported climax recurrence (-25). Factor investigation of the SAI-E) uncovers a comparable construction to that found with the SAI.

CHAPTER 5: MAINSTREAM SOCIETY CAN DESTROY OUR SEXUAL EXPERIENCES

What individual — male or female — hasn't snuck a look at the sensationalist newspapers which line the general store checkout counters? All things considered, they're so in front of you that you can't help it! Be that as it may, tragically, our collaboration with mainstream society can have enduring bad introductions to our sexual experiences. For instance, it's well-known that the media bears much liability regarding taking care of negative self-perception and weaknesses in ladies. Moreover, since ladies' bodies are ceaselessly depicted in profoundly ridiculous ways, it's nothing unexpected that numerous ladies feel shaky in the room since they're estimating themselves against photoshopped norms of "optimal female excellence." And it's quite difficult to feel provocative when you're overpowered by sensations of repugnance about your body!

Yet, the deception doesn't stop at a lady's actual appearance. The female sexual experience is likewise vigorously controlled by the media's message that ladies ought to partake in each sexual position, each underhanded little wrinkle, and each piece of undergarments Victoria's Mystery brings to the table. This creates an extraordinarily unpleasant, difficult situation, notwithstanding, since, in such a case that you truly do partake in the things that are so forcefully pushed on you, you're considered skanky. However, you're bone-chilling or a wet blanket if you don't. Also, assuming you look at the abundance of blended messages that focus on ladies, it becomes apparent that each part of how female sexuality is addressed in the media isn't simply confounding — it's misguided.

Anyway, how might you cleanse your life of these harmful impacts? One special spot to begin is throwing the magazines and praising your excellence. Recognizing that your body, your vagina, and your sentiments are ordinary is a great initial move towards self-acknowledgment. Furthermore, it might likewise assist with knowing that, in 2012, researchers searched through 20 years of examination on the connection between's self-perception and sexual experience and reasoned that your mental self-portrait impacts every part of your sentiments about sex. From excitement to want to your climax, how you feel about your body will decide how great you feel in bed, even down to your readiness to face challenges and open up to your accomplice. Thus, assuming you remove just something single from this part, it ought to be the way that rehearsing self-acknowledgment and further developing your self-perception can, in a real sense, save your sexual coexistence (also your psychological wellness!)

"We'll begin with three center social messages about ladies' sexuality that my understudies wrestle with as their laid out thoughts regarding sex are tested by the science: the ethical message (you are abhorrent), the clinical message (you are unhealthy), and the media message (you are insufficient). Barely anybody completely becomes involved with any of these messages, yet they are there, infringing on our nurseries,"

"On one occasion in class, I read several meanings of "sex resoundingly." First I read from Ideal Marriage: Its Physiology and Method by T. H. van de Velde, from 1926. That's what he composed "typical sex" is that intercourse which happens between two physically mature people of other genders; which prohibits savagery and the utilization of artificial means for delivering curvaceous sensations; which points straightforwardly or by implication at the fulfillment of sexual fulfillment, and which, having accomplished a specific level of excitement, finishes up with the discharge — or emanation — of the semen into the vagina, at the almost synchronous zenith of sensation — or climax — of the two accomplices. Then, at that point, I read from The Hite Report, distributed in 1976, from the section named "Reclassifying Sex": Sex is actual close contact for joy, to impart delight to someone else (or simply alone). You can have intercourse to climax, or not to climax, genital sex, or simply actual closeness — whatever appears acceptable to you. There will never be any motivation to think the "objective" should be intercourse and to attempt to cause what you feel fits into that unique situation. There is no norm of sexual execution "out there" against which you should quantify yourself; you're not managed by "chemicals" or "science." You are allowed to investigate and find your sexuality, to learn or forget anything you need, and to make actual relations with others, of one or the other sex, anything you like."

"The Media Message: "You Are Deficient." Beating, food play, ménages à trois . . . you've done everything, correct? All things considered, you've essentially had clitoral climaxes, vaginal climaxes, uterine climaxes, energy climaxes, expanded climaxes, and various climaxes? Also, you've dominated something like 35 distinct situations for intercourse?"

"What's more, it's playing with our climaxes, pleasure, longing, and sexual fulfillment. There is an immediate compromise between sexual prosperity and self-decisive contemplations about your body. A 2012 survey of 57 examinations, crossing twenty years of exploration, found significant connections between self-perception and pretty much every space of sexual conduct you can envision: excitement, want, climax, recurrence of sex, number of accomplices, sexual self-decisiveness, sexual confidence, utilizing liquor or different medications during sex, participating in unprotected sex, from there, the sky is the limit.

"Proportion of gravity. Look: • Need to shed ten pounds without diet or exercise? Remove your leg at the knee! I ensure, that the following time you step on a scale, you'll weigh less. • Or, hello, need to shed five pounds of fat? Have your cerebrum taken out — its mass is right around 100% fat! • You realize who's in every case slim? Individuals who've been living in a jail camp! • Fast and simple weight reduction! Fly in a plane! Even better, go into space! They don't refer to it as "weightless" for no good reason!"

"Jonathan Haidt and his group have observed that there are six "moral establishments" in the human mind, every one of which is an answer for a specific developmental issue our species has confronted. Of the six, it's the "holiness/corruption" moral establishment I see as generally applicable to sex. The sacredness establishment is about foreign substance aversion, and it's controlled by disdain. People have summed up from evasion of solid impurities (we're naturally sickened by decaying carcasses) to aversion to reasonable pollutants (we can feel nauseated just by the words "spoiling bodies"). You can imagine sacredness as an upward pivot, with defamed and untouchable ways of behaving depicted as "low" and "grimy" and socially endorsed ways of behaving as "high" and "unadulterated." We judge as off-base anything related to lowness. In the Judeo-Christian ethic, bodies are low and soul is high, creature senses are low and human explanation is high, and frequently ladies are low and men are high. Sex attracts consideration down to the base, the creature, the vile, and it, accordingly, triggers the nausea reaction."

"That is the reason sex instructors and sex specialists go through an instructive course of escalated openness, intentionally intended to limit our judgment, disgrace, and loathing responses, so we can answer with open lack of bias to anything understudies or clients bring into the room."

"Openness to media that supports body self-analysis increments body disappointment, negative temperament, low confidence, and, surprisingly, scattered eating. This is maybe most obviously represented by a long-term investigation of the effect of Western media — particularly TV — on young ladies in Fiji. In a culture where there had been "an unmistakable inclination for a strong structure," following three years of openness to late 1990s American TV (think Melrose Spot and Beverly Slopes 90210), the pace of confused eating among teen young ladies rose from 13% to 29 percent, with 74% detailing that they "feel too large or excessively fat," in sharp differentiation to pre-television culture. What's more, this wasn't simply a blip — a decade after the fact, paces of confused eating drifted around 25-30 percent."

"It turns out bad just when you attempt to apply what you picked as appropriate for your sexuality to another person's sexuality."

The finishing-up period of the sexual reaction is the goal. After the climax, the anatomic and physiologic changes of energy switch. In ladies, the orgasmic stage vanishes as vasocongestion reduces, the uterus moves into the genuine pelvis, and the vagina abbreviates and limits. A cloudy sheet of sweat covers the body, and the raised pulse and breath, step by step, get back to business as usual. Assuming climax, there are associative mental vibes of substantial unwinding and sensations of delivery and sexual happiness and fulfillment. Similar physiologic cycles happen at a much slower rate if the climax has not happened. The psychologic reactions are generally either impartial or negative (e.g., proceeded with sexual pressure, frustration at having not experienced climax). As portrayed here, there have not been many endeavors to evaluate the condition of the goal.

Interestingly, some measures survey worldwide assessments of one's sexual life or general fulfillment with sexuality and, like this, mirror a characteristic like perspective on goal. For instance, on the DSFI, there is a 10-thing sexual fulfillment scale. Everything seems to evaluate an alternate part of fulfillment with the sexual life, incorporating fulfillment with the recurrence and scope of sexual exercises, correspondence with an accomplice, the event of climax, and goal sentiments. There is not much psychometric information, yet the accessible data is steady. The inner consistency is .71, and the scale can recognize from physically useless and utilitarian examples.

CHAPTER 6: JUST BECAUSE YOUR GENITALS ARE RESPONDING, IT DOESN'T MEAN YOU'RE AROUSED

On the off chance that you're similar to the vast majority, your accomplice's excitement is presumably one of your number one sections about sex. It feels quite a bit better to realize that you can give them such a lot of joy. In any case, do you have any idea that an actual reaction can, in some cases, be compulsory and doesn't mean your accomplice is stimulated? This is particularly obvious on account of ladies, as studies that estimated bloodstream to the vagina have shown that reading material "excitement reactions" aren't generally a decent sign of your accomplice's fulfillment. In this review, researchers estimated the excitement reactions of all kinds of people while watching obscene recordings. The members were approached to report how stirred they felt at whatever second by turning a dial.

The analysts then found that the connection between their degree of excitement and how much bloodstream to their private parts was half for male members. Yet, for ladies, it was lower than 10%!

Anyway, what might we, at any point, gain from this activity? One important key point may be that assuming you're confounded about whether your female accomplice is partaking as far as you can tell, you should ask her instead of accepting her actual reaction as a prompt. Generally speaking, an excitement reaction in a lady essentially shows that she finds the ongoing boosts physically important. Instead of appreciating it, it could be that her vagina perceives that something is going on in that temperate region of the body and answers appropriately.

This is additionally essential to remember horrible sexual encounters like assault. For instance, numerous survivors feel culpability or disgrace because their vagina answered while they were being attacked. Many even trusts this implies that they "merited" or "needed" it when that is certainly not the situation. In like manner, numerous men feel disgrace since they unexpectedly become stimulated while seeing an assault scene in a film. Yet, this shouldn't continue causing pointless activity for men or women. In the two cases, your reaction is nothing unusual or dishonorable.

Similarly, as you can exhibit an exciting reaction during a consensual encounter you're despising, the equivalent is valid for non-consensual sex acts. Assuming your body automatically answers by seeing or getting sexual improvements, it doesn't imply that you're a terrible individual, that you need to be attacked, or that you must cause sexual brutality to other people. All things considered, your body is answering in a way that doesn't have anything to do with your actual sentiments.

"What this exploration proposes is that a lady's close-to-home experience is bound to agree with her look and her vocal expression, while a man's encounter is bound to agree with his pulse and bloodstream."

"Each person, eventually in his life, has the experience of needing sex, needing an erection, and the erection simply isn't there. At that time, the erection (or absence of erection) isn't a proportion of his advantage — he could try and awaken the exceptionally next morning with an erection when it's only a bother."

"Genital reaction, which occurs between your legs, is anticipating. Excitement, which occurs between your ears, incorporates appreciating."

"In this way, E. L. James, if you understand this: Oil implies it was physically significant, which enlightens us nothing concerning whether it was physically engaging. Subsequently, I unassumingly demand that in the following release, Dark tells Ana, "Feel this. Perceive how physically pertinent your body thinks about actual contact with your hindquarters and privates, Anastasia. That gives me no data about whether you enjoyed it. Did you like it? No? Twofold poo, let me make it dependent upon you by perusing Emily Nagoski's book about ladies' sexual prosperity, so I have an idea sometime later." Much obliged."

"If that is valid, when your primary care physician taps your knee's patellar ligament and your leg throws out, that should mean you need to kick your PCP. Or on the other hand, when you have a hypersensitive response to dust, you should stand blossoms. Or on the other hand, when your mouth waters around a significant piece of rotten, wounded peach, you should think that it is delectable."

"Try not to misunderstand me — you should kick your PCP and you could loathe blossoms and you could appreciate rotten, wounded peaches. Yet, your programmed physiological cycles are not how we would know that. No. Programmed physiological cycles are, ya know, programmed, not earnest."

"This carries me to a sentence each undergrad who takes an exploration strategies class will remember: "Connection doesn't suggest causation." It alludes to the cum hoc consequently proper hoc paradox — "with this, subsequently along these lines" — and that implies that since two things happen together doesn't imply that one thing caused the other thing."

"The quintessential model in the twenty-first century is the connection among privateers and a dangerous atmospheric deviation. This is a joke made by Bobby Henderson, as a feature of the conviction arrangement of the Congregation of the Flying Spaghetti Beast. Henderson needed to have a point about the effect of causation and relationship, so he drew a chart that plotted an expansion in worldwide temperature with the sharp drop in the number of nautical privateers. Did the deficiency of privateers cause worldwide environmental change?"

Want: Really, It's anything but A Drive

"If sex were a drive, similar to food hunger, the 30% of ladies who once in a long while or never experience an unconstrained craving for sex are . . . all things considered, what might we call an individual who never experienced unconstrained crave food, regardless of whether she hadn't eaten in days or weeks or months? That individual is certainly wiped out! If sex is a yearning and you never get eager, something is off about You. What's more, when you accept something isn't quite right about you, your pressure reaction kicks in. What's more, when your pressure reaction kicks too, your greatest advantage in sex vanishes (for the vast majority). Demanding that sex is a drive is telling a solid individual with a responsive craving that she's debilitated — say it frequently enough and in the long run, she'll trust you. Also, when she trusts you, unexpectedly it's valid. The concern makes individuals wiped out."

"It's your basis speed being unsatisfied. At the end of the day, it's not the way that you feel . . . it's how you feel about how you feel."

"What I like most about interest as a similarity to sex is that it implies your accomplice is not a creature to be pursued for food, but a mysterious guardian whose secret profundities are endless. Sexual fatigue can happen provided that you're presently not inquisitive."

"The two of them are — depending, I think, on how you conceptualize "want." Recall section 3, the differentiation between enthusiasm and appreciation. For Perel, want is enthusiasm. Needing. Looking for. Hankering. The error diminishes the quest for an objective, to place it in heartfelt terms. Furthermore, Gottman and the couples in the examination he refers to, want more to do with getting a charge out. Holding. Enjoying. Permitting. Investigating this second together, seeing what it is endlessly similar to it. Assuming you'll permit a food similitude, Perel's style is about hunger as the mystery ingredient that makes a feast flavorful. Gottman's is tied in with getting back from work and preparing supper with your accomplice, having a glass of wine while you cook, taking care of one another every one of the strawberries you intended to save for dessert, then, at that point, plunking down together and relishing each significant piece. In the Perel style, you come to join forces with your fire previously stirred up. In the Gottman style, you stir up one another's fire."

"In season 2 of the Canadian television series Slings and Bolts, theater chief Geoffrey Tennant mentors a couple of youthful entertainers battling to play Romeo and Juliet. He advises them to run as quickly as possible around the block, pursuing one another, then irregularly do push-ups while enthusiastically painting as they would prefer through the text of the overhang scene. "Juliet's" evaluation of how this procedure changes her appreciation for the text: "Wow it's simply . . . enthusiastic, it's. . . truly wonderful, yet it's, truth be told, um, sexual, as well," she wheezes."

"Methodology 1: Stuff That Raises Your Pulse."

"Methodology 2: Significant Difficulties."

CHAPTER 7: EUPHORIA FOR EVERYONE, THE AWESOME REWARD FOR THE CLIMAX

The most pleasurable climaxes happen when all aspects of you are available and working together in the quest for one shared objective: happiness.

Meta-Feelings: A definitive Sex-Good Setting

"Yet, maybe the greatest test is that when the guide and the landscape don't coordinate, our cerebrums attempt to make the guide valid, constraining our experience into the state of the guide. "No, no, this is the path," we say as we stagger through the shrubbery. "It expresses so on the guide."

"At the point when the guide (the content) doesn't appear to fit the territory (your experience), the guide is off-base, not the landscape. • Everybody's territory and everybody's guide are not quite the same as every other person's."

"What these two principles mean is that your best wellspring of information about your sexuality is your own inside experience. Whenever you notice a conflict between the landscape and the guide — and everybody does, sooner or later — consistently expect your body is correct. Furthermore, accepting everybody's body is unique to yours — similar to everybody's guides. And that implies everybody's excursion from lost voyager to dominate guide will be unique."

"We're an illustration of how even hereditarily indistinguishable nurseries, planted with very much like seeds, may, in any case, develop into totally different landscapes. It turns out she has a somewhat more touchy brake than I do, and I have a somewhat more delicate gas pedal. So maybe the Media Message was a somewhat better fit for my local sexuality and the Ethical Message a somewhat better fit for Amelia's, thus various thoughts flourished and developed."

"I used to believe that it was the consciousness of your inward express that made a difference, yet in many examinations, "perception" of the inside state is not a critical indicator of prosperity. No, the best meta-feeling indicator of prosperity is a variable known as "nonjudge.""

RITA J. ALEXANDER

CONCLUSION: YOU ARE THE MYSTERIOUS FIXING

Our lives are, in many cases, directed by normal misinterpretations about sex, which can prompt a lot of tension and disarray. For instance, many individuals stress that their vagina is unusually molded, not encountering the "right" levels of excitement, or that their sex drive is excessively low. However, our bodies are more perplexing than we've been persuaded to think, and the media is liable for taking care of our frailties and misconceptions. Truth be told, vaginas arrive in different shapes and varieties, and there's no such thing as a "sex drive."

Rather, this is a typical misinterpretation because we classify sex as a need like food or sanctuary and accept, at least for now, that we're persuaded to seek after it by a developmental "drive." However, sex is a craving as opposed to something we want to get by, which implies that we don't have a "sex drive", even a bunch of gas pedals and breaks. The speed with which we get into stuff or ram on the breaks relies upon a wide assortment of upgrades not entirely set in stone by setting. In this way, whether your setting includes the progression of time, the new birth of a kid, or a huge measure of pressure, it's vital to realize that your reaction is typical and it's OK on the off chance that you're not in the mindset at present. It's likewise commonplace to be delayed in answering any sexual feeling, which doesn't mean something isn't quite right about you. All things being equal, you could just need some additional time, additional foreplay, or the capacity to gradually warm up to sexual sentiments through the movement of a heartfelt environment and cozy discussion.

You ought to likewise recollect that pressure and media portrayal essentially affect the sexual experiences of people the same. Since sensations of pressure or disappointment with our bodies can rapidly kill the state of mind, it's justifiable on the off chance that you want time to rehearse self-acknowledgment and cycle through the pressure interaction before you're ready to have pleasant intercourse. Yet, regardless of what you battle with, Nagoski welcomes perusers to recollect that everybody is allowed to develop and investigate their sexuality.

"We live in a Main 5 Hints world, where there are twelve new strategies for marvelous fellatio every month, trailed by six hot new positions he's for a long while been itching to attempt. This world is brimming with fun, invigorating, engaging things that draw and hold our consideration. Yet, the construction of the fact of the matter is calmer, slower, more private, and thus significantly more fascinating than simple diversion. What's more, it lives solely inside you, in the calm snapshots of bliss, in the jostling snapshots of stress, in the torn minutes when the herd that is you is attempting all the while to take off from danger and toward delight."

"Side effects, nor were they more mindful of their inside state — the "notice" factor. Not a chance. Individuals who were less affected by their side effects were the people who were nonjudging! At the end of the day, it isn't the side effects that foresee how much nervousness upsets an individual's life, it's the way an individual feels about those side effects. It's not the way that you feel — it's not in any event, monitoring how you feel. It's how you feel about how you feel. Also, individuals who feel nonjudging about their sentiments improve."

"Feeling instructing instructs you that • You can perceive lower force feelings so you can oversee them before they heighten. •

Pessimistic feelings are a characteristic reaction to pessimistic life-altering situations. Since pessimistic life-altering situations are now and again inescapable, gloomy feelings are as well. • Because gloomy feelings are an ordinary piece of life, they are examined, given names, and sympathized with. "It's generally expected that occasionally it feels hard," "When you feel awful, we love you similarly as much as when you feel better," and "You cry all you want to, honey." Your pity, outrage, and dread are indications of being human."

"Feeling excusing, then again, instructs you that sentiments aren't a passage, they're a cavern . . . with a stream of cyanide . . . what's more, 1,000 rodents . . . in obscurity. Where you'll be caught for eternity. So anything you do, KEEP OUT."

"In any case, awkward sentiments occur. They are the ordinary, solid reaction to negative life-altering situations. At the point when you experience unfairness, outrage occurs. At the point when you experience misfortune, bitterness occurs. At the point when you experience impediments in your advancement toward an objective, dissatisfaction occurs. At the point when you experience a danger, dread occurs. Also, regardless of whether you just expect any of these things, you might just experience the inclination, and it will be similarly basically as awkward as though the thing were occurring."

"There's no reason for feeling it." Indeed, there is. The purpose of feeling an inclination you can't hope to make a difference with is to allow it to release and complete the cycle so it can end."

"All I can tell you," I said, "is that all that you're encountering, every one of the problematic sentiments and all the aggravation, is an ordinary piece of the mending system. Everybody goes through it unexpectedly, and it's impossible to know how long it will endure. It sucks for some time, and afterward step by step it improves. In any case, I can let you know this without a doubt: Every survivor I've at any point known has tracked down their direction through it."

"Neither of you picked your sentiments — yet both of you pick how you feel about those sentiments."

"Sentiments aren't hazardous . . . however they can be utilized perilously. One of the focal messages in feeling excusing meta-feelings is that sentiments are intrinsically perilous — harmful and frightful to yourself and the individuals around you. Individuals might trust this on the off chance that they experienced childhood in our current reality where individuals utilized sentiments to harm or control others — and utilizing your sentiments to purposely hurt individuals is contrary to the guidelines. Generally significant: You're not permitted to utilize your sentiments to harm or control yourself! (Self-sympathy!) Nor are you permitted to utilize them to harm or control your accomplice or others — and others, including your accomplice, aren't permitted to utilize them against you, all things considered."

"This is pretty much exacting: It's not the way that you feel (torment). It's how you feel (open-minded or not) about how you feel."

"Human experience, that what's on our guide is equivalent to what is on others' guides. "All of us are simply attempting to have a place someplace." We need to realize that we are protected inside the limits of shared Recollect what Claudie expressed way back in chapter 2: have a place. I believe that to feel typical is to feel that you. For what reason is ordinary the objective? What truly do individuals truly need when they need to be ordinary?"

"Lastly, she turned out to be a lot gentler with herself when she saw herself being self-basic about her body or having a blameworthy outlook on joy. She didn't share with herself, "Stop it!" She recently thought, "Correct. There are the self-decisive considerations once more." She rehearsed nonjudgment."

"It's not the way that you feel. It's how you feel about how you feel."

www.ingramcontent.com/pod-product-compliance
Lightning Source LLC
Chambersburg PA
CBHW051715250726
48653CB00007B/3049